I0415537

Anal Sex

By Jennifer S.

Copyright (C) 2014

ISBN-13: 978-1491216675
ISBN-10: 1491216670

Erotic BDSM Books - Your Erotic BDSM Book Publisher
EroticBDSMbooks.com

This book comes with four additional bonus books. Your books are presented in this order:

1) **Anal Sex**..**3**
2) The Absolutely Essential Guide to Erotic Breast Massage........**18**
3) Special Things To Do During 3 Hours of Sex; A Step-by-step Guide..**26**
4) THE PS-SPOT ORGASM: Women Don't Wait Any Longer For This Kind of Pleasure..**34**
5) Absolutely Essential Tips for Buying & Selling On eBay............**49**

Book 1

Anal Sex - 14 Male - Female Anal Sex Scenes

1. My name is Erica. I'm a 114 lb pretty Mexican lady with straight black hair and full lips. My breast size is 32C. I was particularly proud of my firm very well proportioned ass that was perfect for playing with, and other things.

It was the morning on the 16th of December and as is the norm on weekdays I got on a very crowded subway to go to work. I was wearing a short black dress. I had black stockings on as well as black bra and panties. It was winter so I also wore a coat.

I was lucky enough to catch the express train even though it was packed. Nearly 15 minutes into the 45 minute ride I felt something brush against my ass as I stood holding onto the rail in the middle of the subway car. Then it happened again. Touching my ass is a huge turn on for me and I was still sleepy so I not only didn't get concerned about it but actually got turned on by it. Still I had forgotten about it when it happened a 3rd time. It was so crowded but I still tried turning around. I got a glimpse of a great looking guy looking down on me and standing right behind me. I knew it was him. He had a tie on and looked like an executive. He had a friendly but firm face. Then he leaned against my butt and now I was feeling his cock inside his pants. Suddenly the subway car went into a turn that forced my ass further into the cock. Suddenly I felt nothing and for the next 5 minutes I was horny as hell just thinking about what had just happened. If there was room I wanted to turn around and see what happened to him but what if he was gone and there was someone else there? What if I thought it was him but it was somebody else. I was very nervous but really turned on. Nothing like this had ever happened to me before.

Suddenly, a man whispered in my ear to stay still, not make a sound, and enjoy it. Soon I felt a hand sliding over my so spankable ass, slowly working its way down and under my skirt, targeting my panties. Fingers went inside my panties and down the crack of my ass to my asshole. The next thing I knew my asshole was being taken by a lubricated finger, a long one too. The finger rammed my anus and stopped me right in my tracks. I was so turned on I didn't want to turn around or say anything that could interfere with this adventure, besides I love to have my asshole played with as much as I love to get taken in it.

My ass was being finger fucked by a pro for seemingly an eternity. He was very deliberate. He started out slowly then took me very fast then rested with slow thrusts and went back to fast pumping. Oh my gosh, what if I came right there in the subway car! Fortunately it was so crowded and loud that if I was quiet nobody was likely to even notice, but suddenly it stopped and his delicious finger had partially been taken out of my ass. I stood there hoping for more, then, before I could turn around, my invader suddenly drove his finger in as far as it could go and left it there for the remainder of the ride, wiggling it regularly.

It was the most exciting subway ride I've ever had. While his finger rested inside of me I decided to try and cum. I closed my eyes and inconspicuously fucked his finger and sure enough had a nice, quiet orgasm as I held tight to the overhead rail so I wouldn't fall incase my knees buckled.

Then as we approached a stop, I felt his finger pull out of me. I wanted to turn around in case he wanted to get to know me better but was too shy to.

I arrived at the office and was horny the entire day. Later that evening I put my two vibrators to very good and lengthy use.

Every day I got on the subway at the same time looking for him. It was frustrating in a sense, but I really wondered what he was like and fantasized about having a date with him. Was he a great lover? Would he only want to take me in my ass?

I had given up on finding what in my mind I had somehow made into my dream man, when a week later I got on the subway to work and there he was. The subway wasn't as crowded then and even though I relished the thought of him finger fucking my ass again, it would be tougher to hid, besides there was an open seat next to him so I sat there. Would this be my only chance to get to know him better?

I couldn't ask him if he was the guy that played with my asshole, what if he wasn't. He could also be afraid to admit to it as he may be afraid he could get in trouble. He wasn't starting the conversation so I worked up the courage and asked him for the time. He was friendly and gave it to me and thankfully the conversation developed. We even agreed to meet for drinks later that day but my ass being finger fucked hadn't yet come up.

Well anyway I now live with him and yes that was him. Now he enjoys my ass in many other ways and whenever he wants it.

----

2. My boyfriend doesn't like to fuck me in the ass a real lot. I on the other hand love it in the ass. Therefore, I got pretty excited when Kevin called and said he was coming over to take me in the ass and I shouldn't have anything on, have had an enema and be on the bed waiting for him. How nice, tonight I would have a little delicious pain and A LOT of pleasure.

90 minutes or so later he arrived. He had a key to my apartment so he walked right into the bedroom where I was eagerly waiting for him. His cloths were off in a flash and he sat down in front of me on the bed where I eagerly sucked on his cock. After 5 minutes of sucking, he lifted my head off of him and told me to get on my hands and knees. He lubed himself up, then entered my very ready ass.

"Does it hurt?" Kevin asked me, sliding another couple inches into me. I replied by shoving my ass back against him and taking the rest of his pulsing cock into my tight hole. His moans of pleasure told me that he was enjoying it too. He cautiously began pumping his cock in and out. I could tell he was concerned about hurting me and even though it did hurt some, I'm the impatient type, and started pushing myself back into him, getting him to fuck me harder and faster. "Ooh yes" he said. "I'm going to cum in your tight little ass!"

That comment sent me over the edge, and I orgasmed long and hard. Just as I was finishing, I felt splashes of hot cum shooting deep inside my ass. It felt amazing, and it made me cum again.

Well this now has become a regular part of our playtime.

----

3. It was my boyfriend's birthday, and as well as a gift of a great shirt, I decided to give him another more personal present, my ass.

My name is Cindy and I'm a 29 year old brunette. 125 lbs, 5'3", 38B boobs. Brad and I had been dating for a couple of months. He wanted to take me in my ass but I resisted it as I'd never experienced such a thing before. He had put toys in my ass when playing with me, and often when he was taking my pussy doggie style he would also put a dildo in it. Thus when he thrust into me, his pelvis pushed both his cock into my pussy as well as the dildo into my ass. It was great to be on my hands and knees with both of my holes being filled!

A few days ahead of time I told him on the phone about the special birthday present I was giving him, and I must admit that the anticipation was killing me. I couldn't wait. If I liked it I'd want us to do it a lot more often.

The night arrived and after a small birthday gathering at a bar, we returned for the main event.

Our clothes were off in a flash. I told him how I just couldn't wait for him to take me in my ass and how I had been thinking about it all week. He thought this would be a very memorable birthday present.

With my pussy at the edge of the bed, he ate it like it was dessert. With his birthday present in mind I gifted him with lots of pussy juice. He then told me to get further up on the bed and get on my elbows and knees. The moment was not far off. He then lubed my anus up, pushing the lubrication deep and spending a lot of time finger fucking me. Little did he know how ready I was for this anal treat. He then sat against the head board and had me lay down on my stomach in front of him and make his cock hard with my mouth. I sucked away on his cock, sucking down his ooze as I made his cock harder and harder. I loved to feel a cock hardening in my mouth and clearly he was really enjoying himself too. Then suddenly he lifted my head off of his cock. The moment of truth had arrived.

He got behind me and oh my god I got entered! He started pumping my ass in a slow and deliberate motion. Like I envisioned all week. I loosened my anus as much as I could, and that seemed to make all the difference in the world. I figured I'd enjoy finally being taken in the ass and even if it took several minutes, I did! I guess it helps to be so turned on.

Well that was a while back and being taken in the ass is a regular occurrence now. When we're having sex, Tom starts in my pussy and finishes in my ass!

----

4. The long and short of it is that I screwed up and accepted that my husband had the right to punish me. I would have preferred the usual spanking but he's done that so much with me over the years that mainly it just turns me on, so he thought of another punishment. I would have to wear a butt plug all day. He would put it on before we went to work and after we both got home he would take it out, at a time of his choosing. (We work at the same place in the garment district in Los Angeles. We had good jobs thanks to it being his family's business.)

He had put butt plugs in me before at different times for significant periods, such as when I was doing housework. Only on one other occasion however did I leave the house with a butt plug in me. It was once when I drove to the supermarket, with a stopover at the gas station for a fill-up, (of gas that is.)

I would have protested but I didn't know what other nasty punishment he would then do to me instead. (He can be very mischievous when it comes to punishing me.)

A very important part of this punishment was going to be which butt plug I would have to "wear". We had several. We had one he called the "spreader". It was 5 inches long and 1½ inches at its thickest point. There was one that was 6 inches long and an inch at its thickest. It looked like a penis and vibrated (mmmmm.) There is also the butt plug he called "ole reliable." It was 4 1/2" long and tapers to 1" at its widest. Then there were the anal beads. (As you can tell my asshole gets a lot of attention when it comes to sex.) He chose one of the sets of anal beads.

Tomorrow would be Wednesday and that was determined to be the fateful day. Tomorrow came along and he picked my clothes out for me. I would be wearing a dark brown skirt, one of my stronger pairs of white panties (with an extra one in my purse just in case,) a white bra and a white button down blouse.

With just my bra on I put on my make-up then bent over a chair and waited as my husband came over, lubed me a bit and inserted the anal beads well into my ass. Then using lots of white cloth first aid tape, he taped my asshole securely shut. After a quick spanking, we continued getting ready for work and I got in the car with him (often we take separate cars but not today as he was having too much fun watching me fidget in my seat.)

I would be allowed to lubricate my anus as much as I wanted throughout the day, but I never did. If I was sitting I could pivot into a comfortable position. The bending down to sit could really get my attention. Getting up and walking was a different story and as the day progressed it made for some interesting moments.

Twice my husband called me down to the warehouse where he worked, to watch me walk. When no one was watching he had me bend over with my butt in front of him. Bending over was something I had to be very careful doing as the dildo stuck out a bit that way, even though my muscles, the tape and my underwear mostly kept it in place. He had fun pushing it in even though it would quickly pop back towards him a bit. It also got me so turned on.

Still my anus felt raw after we got home and my husband finally took it out. But the sex that night was mind blowing!

----

5. I was on my hands and knees and Tom was kneeling behind me.

I found myself saying "Oh yes! I want more of you in me. I want you to finger fuck me like I've never been fucked before." I felt Tom slide yet another finger inside my pussy, then, without warning his lubricated, well manicured thumb entered my tight ass. I cried out and began bucking my hips against his hand. It hurt a bit but oh it felt so good.

"Oh god, fuck me hard." I felt Tom rocking his hand back and forth and up and down. First his fingers thrust into my pussy then his hand pulled out and up so his thumb could thrust even further into my ass. He pumped his finger in my ass all the while fucking my pussy with his other fingers. "Oh god yes! That feels so good!"

"What am I doing to you baby? Tell me."

"You're fucking my pussy with your fingers, and fucking my ass with your thumb."

Just then, Tom pulled out a finger that was in my pussy and also stuck it in my ass along with his thumb. Then he furiously fucked both my holes. "Now you've got two fingers in my ass. Yes please, fuck me harder! Faster!"

I felt myself tightening up and Tom must have felt it also as he fucked my pussy and ass hard after slowing a bit for a rest. I exploded onto his hand and began bucking my hips against him. The orgasm I had was so intense, I heard myself ask him to stop, but I didn't mean it. I moaned and screamed, and suddenly I came again. In time Tom pulled his hand out of both my holes.

All I could do was lay there, completely exhausted. "Did you enjoy that baby?" Tom asked softly.

"Mmmmmmmmmmmmmmmmmmmmmm" I replied as Tom kissed me tenderly before walking away.

----

6. My husband bought me a fucking machine for Christmas. It was an amazing surprise that I never expected. He goes on the road a significant amount so for that reason alone it would come in handy. Needless to say it got used often, which doesn't help our electricity bill!

One night though it was used on me for something unexpected, for punishment. I had forgotten to pay some bills which caused some problems to our credit rating. It was just a case of being forgetful and my husband wanted to nip that in the bud.

That night, at dinner, he informed me that my punishment tonight would be to be taken in the ass by the spanking machine, and only in the ass. We had tried anal sex before but I found it hurt too much but after screwing up our credit rating I found myself in no position to argue, and if anything felt I needed to be punished.

An hour or so after dinner, Jim told me to strip and wait for him next to the machine. I was really nervous and even trembled from time to time. I knew Jim wanted to take me in my ass more often but it hurt, besides I exercised my pussy good and hard to make sure it was nice and tight for him.

Soon he came over and told me to "assume the position". I got on my elbows and knees at the usual spot and distance from the machine's arm that had the dildo at its end.

He didn't waste anytime either. He slowly slid the machine's dildo up into my ass. Even though it was thoroughly lubricated, it took a bit of time before it was finally stuffed all the way up my ass. I tried to ignore it and I hoped I would find it more comfortable later on. He then got up and went to the kitchen to get a drink.

When he came back I knew the time had come. There is a manual control lever on the fucking machine so one can manually make the machine's arm go back and forth; he activated that and my ass began to officially be taken.

He started slow and it made me moan. It did hurt some but starting slow like this was real helpful. I put my head down and loosen my asshole as much as I could.

What I really wanted to be able to do is cum from it. Also I knew that Jim at some point would sit in front of me and I'd be sucking on his cock while my ass was being taken.

"Keep your butt in place" he ordered. I didn't realize it but I was moving out of place some so less and less of the dildo was entering me. I quickly straighten out. Then Jim let the machine take over by turning it on and setting it to automatic.

The noise of the machine startled me but that ended up being a momentary concern. The fact is that fucking my ass was indirectly working my clit and maybe my A-spot.

The good news is that I was feeling okay and things would get better still as suddenly I heard the unmistakable humming of a vibrator next to me. Jim ran the vibrator along my pussy slowly then more quickly, and that would be the end of my fear of being taken anally!

"Oh yes, please, more..." Was that me that said that? Wow, it was. I actually was now humping the fucking machine and felt my first orgasm coming on. "Ohhhhhhhhh." I put my head down and just hollered, "Oh god yes...more..." I came all over that vibrator and know my ass being fucked had a lot to do with it.

Jim then took away the vibrator and told me I had to cum from the ass fucking alone. I wanted so much to do that and knew

I could. He got in front of me and sure enough I was sucking on his cock while my ass was being taken by the machine. It was amazing. He reached down and played with my boobs too. I now had two of my holes filled and my boobs being played with, but still no orgasm. 10 or so minutes later I was not only rewarded for all my sucking efforts with a mouth full of my husband's cum but I also came along with him as well!

Well I now often get taken by the fucking machine like that night, sometimes in my pussy, sometimes in my ass and sometimes in my pussy and then ass. Assuming my husband's home during that time I usually have his cock in my mouth, sucking the daylights out of it.

What a punishment that turned out to be!

----

7. After my boyfriend Joe spends some time fucking my pussy, it's time to take me in my ass. As part of foreplay he has already lubed my tight hole. He slowly puts his cock into my very tight asshole. It feels so tight going in and can hurt for a while. Sometimes Joe fucks my ass really fast and sometimes he starts slow. I'll be moaning or crying out the whole time. During that time I play with my clit and/or use a vibrator on my wet pussy. I fuck my pussy with my hand while Joe fucks my ass. His thrusts are very deep and very hard. Joe will spank me while taking me in my ass. It stings but feels so good.

----

8. After watching TV in bed, my husband and I decide to fuck, so we take off the rest of our clothes. After I suck on his cock to make it hard, my husband tells me to get on my hands and knees. He then guides his very hard, thick cock into my dripping wet cunt. He thrusts deeper and deeper and it feels so incredible.

Soon his hands are all over my boobs and I turn my head and lean back so we can kiss deeply and passionately. He grabs my ass and starts to spank it, first lightly but the swats keep getting harder and harder and that feels great too. No words are usually spoken while we are lost in our hot, wild sex.

At some point my husband reaches for the lube and applies it to my tight hole, who's turn to be taken has come. He slowly glides his cock into my ass. I gasp at first from the delicious pain but he takes his time. At first he enters me slowly, but soon really starts to fuck my tight ass. He spanks my cheeks which make them sore but it feels great to be spanked while I'm being fucked in the ass. The thrusts are so deep and while he is fucking my sweet ass I am fucking my pussy with my fingers. I'm so wet that my pussy cums all over my fingers. I then take my fingers out of my wet cunt and let my husband taste them. He licks all the cum up and continues to fuck my ass harder and faster. Eventually he cums in my ass with a shout.

----

9. I love to ride Craig while Jon fucks me in the ass. I didn't like ass play until recently but I gave into their persistent requests as they told me they would be gentle and make me love it by the time we're finished. I start by straddling Craig and ride him with abandon. My pussy gets soaking wet as I ride him up and down. I then I push my ass up into the air and Jon lubes my tight ass and his cock. He slowly puts his first few inches into my ass. It feels different and hurts for a while, but I'm so turned on that I don't feel it that much. He begins pushing more and more and now he is all the way into my tight ass. Oh my God, it feels amazing. Throughout all this I continue to fuck Craig. With two cocks now securely in me, I start to cum. "Oh god I'm going to cum" I scream. I cum as their cocks pound my pussy and ass.

In time we decide to switch. Jon cleans himself off well from having been in my ass and puts on a new condom. We would now stand up and I would get fucked like a sandwich. As I'm standing, Jon kind of holds me up and Craig does the same as it's now Craig's turn to fuck me in the ass. (As noted they use condoms and clean up before entering my pussy if previously been in my ass.) It was so different, bizarre, wild and dirty! As I'm cumming I tell them that I want to be their naughty slut who loves to suck and fuck.

Wow, I can feel their cocks bump against eachother from time to time through my flesh. Suddenly the testosterone really kicks in and they get into a competition to see who can fuck me in the hole they're in the hardest and fastest. We are like animals. What fun we are having. The sweat is pouring off our bodies and we are groaning and moaning like wild beasts. Gosh knows how many calories we burning! My pussy is dripping and all the friction feels great.

----

10. My husband spent over an hour last night playing with my anus. He wants to take me there but I think it's a sin so I say no, but he's so persistent so I agreed to let him play with it as long as he wants, as long as he doesn't take me there with his penis.

Well he now plays with my anus often using his fingers and sex toys. Last night was for the longest time by far.

Last night he sat on chair (we call it "the chair") in the middle of the room and told me to lay over his lap, like I would be if I was getting a spanking. We're both naked. Next to him on the right is small table. On it is what he'll use on me. It has the lube, sex toys (the use of which I don't think is a sin), towel to wipe me and/or himself off with and anything he is going to spank me with like paddles, a strap and sometimes even a hairbrush!

First though, after I was done cleaning up from dinner, we went into the bedroom and I gave him a long massage. As is norma,l we were both naked. While I massage him, he plays with my breasts. I love it when he does that.

Finally it was time for me to use my mouth on his penis so he could have an orgasm. I laid down on my side and sucked away, feeling his cock get harder and harder in my mouth. It wouldn't be long before he filled my mouth with his seed.

We rested for a while then he told me it was time for us to go to the "chair". My husband just loves to play with my asshole. It took me a while to get used to it but now I really enjoy it.

I lay over his lap. He massaged my butt and legs then tells me to spread my legs. He then uses a vibrator on my vagina until I have an orgasm. It was so nice. But that was just the beginning. I then get a spanking with two of the paddles. During the spanking he'd use the vibrator on me again, often I can orgasm from just that but for some reason I couldn't last night. Then it was time for my anus to be played with, and it would be played with for a very long time!

After that we go back to the bedroom for intercourse.

----

11. My 34th birthday was one I will not forget. My fiancée promised me a special and unusual birthday and that is certainly what I got.

We've been together for almost two years. Our sexual interests have evolved a good deal. One of the things that's developed is our interest in anal sex. Now, when we have sex, Jack starts in my pussy and finishes in my ass.

Ok, so after my birthday party, we were alone.

We kissed and cuddled on the couch for a while then Jack told me to go to the bedroom, strip, get on the bed and wait for my birthday surprise, which I did.

As he was about to enter the room he told me to close my eyes. I heard him enter and felt a bunch of stuff get dumped onto the bed in front of me. He said I could open my eyes and low and behold, sitting in front of me were a dozen brand new anal sex toys still in their wrappers! Jack told me that most were going to get used on me tonight!

First I was scared and started to feel a tightness in my stomach, though also a throbbing between my legs. I bet I got wet then and there.

I looked the toys over. There were two anal trainer kits, couple of "lube shooters" to get the lube in all the way, 2 rump shakers, 6 butt plugs of various sizes, a vibrating anal probe, 3 sets of anal beads, all sorts of exotic lubes, a black throbbing anal balloon that gets inserted and inflated to stay securing in an ass, another expandable butt plug, 2 fingered butt plugs, an anal dilator kit and an oversized flesh colored butt plug that looked like trouble.

Well guess what we did nightly for some time! It was a blast, though sometimes I would need a few of nights off for my asshole to regroup. After that night Jack would regularly play with my ass with one or more of the anal toys, then we would make love.

Ladies what are you getting for your birthday?

14

12. You cover my eyes with a blindfold and tell me to bend over the back of the couch so my naked ass is in the air. I hear you moving behind me but don't know what to expect until I feel one of your lubricated fingers probing my tight little hole. You insert another wet finger which I can't help but start fucking. With your free hand you slap my ass hard and tell me to stay still. Then you remove your fingers and I feel another pressure against my hole. It's bigger than your fingers and I realize that it's a butt plug, and from the feel of it one of the largest you have ever used on me. I want to pull away but know that wouldn't be right so I brace myself as you slide it in, which you do gently at first until the initial resistance of my muscles has passed, then you push hard so your full length is in me. I moan again at this intrusion.

I hear a noise and realize that you inserted an inflatable butt plug and now you're inflating it. You inflate it past the point of comfort but I keep quiet. You then attach both of my hands together with handcuffs. You then tie ropes around each of my ankles which spread my legs good and wide. You then tie each of my ankles to opposite couch legs so my holes are on display for all to see. I am now immobile with my pussy and asshole sticking out very invitingly, even though my ass is full. Then you turn and leave the room. I am now alone and scared but I've been like this before so I start to feel a familiar tightness in my stomach and that wetness between my legs. I know that you will return and fuck me to your heart's content. Each thrust you make into me will also pound up against the inflated butt plug in me. While you're taking me you will reach down and play with my tits at will. I will cum so hard for you.

----

13. She said her name was Carla but who knows. She charged me $50 to fuck her in the ass. I never saw signs of STDs on her but again who knows. She would come over to my apartment, strip and jerk me off until I was hard. (Sometimes, unfortunately she would first go into the bathroom and snort cocaine before sex which was really uncool.) After she got me hard she would put a condom on me, lubed me up real good and get on her hands and knees, or elbows and knees. I didn't need to be particularly gentle

15

in taking her in her ass and could slide right in and fuck hard within seconds. She loved it too. She would play with her clit with her hand and/or a vibrator. I'd spank her butt too as she'd start begging for that after a while.

She'd give me up to 20 minutes of ass fucking (I only fucked her in her pussy once but it was too loose and frankly I was pissed she even made me pay money for that.)

If I hadn't cum within 20 minutes, I'd pull out and she would lube my dick up even more and masturbate me to orgasm, which she was really good at actually.

Anyway, I heard she got busted for prostitution and hoped it wasn't anything worse. What sucked was I was afraid that the cops had gotten pictures of me with her or something, which fortunately they hadn't.

Anyway I really miss that tight ass and how much she enjoyed being fucked in it. I've fucked two ladies since but both wouldn't let me fuck their ass, which really sucks.

----

14. I'm a 36 year old white female that's been fucked in the ass many times. The first two times I was drunk which may be the best way to get acquainted with getting it in the ass.

I have a fuck buddy that loves fucking me in the ass. It was the first time for him and I think he hardly can believe his luck, not only am I a pretty no-commitment fuck buddy but I love it up the ass also.

Well he did something the other night that blew me away. He called and told me to clean out my asshole really well (which I do before sex anyway.) He seemed really serious about it so I enemaed and soaped and did all the cleaning I could. Something was going on here as he was never like this. I also had to wonder if he wasn't freaking out in terms of thinking I was a dirty slut or something of that nature. That would be a hassle if I had to find another fuck buddy but doable as I went through dieting hell to get down to a size 6.

Anyway he came over to my place and we had the usual chit chat, watched American Idol and retired to my room when my nosey roommate came home.

Our clothes were off in a jiffy and wow did I ever have a treat, he ate out my asshole, as in with his mouth, and not for a minute or two but for 20-30 minutes!

He tongue fucked me several times throughout it all, often he played with my clit during all this.

I had never had this done to me and after I got over the surprise, I realized how excited I was. Fortunately I had 2 different vibrators within arm's reach and I put them to quick use on and in my pussy. My orgasms were amazing.

Girls if you're into anal sex you've got to experience this. Warning to the guys, tongue fucking an asshole for a long time can really make your tongue sore!

THE END

Book #2 - The Absolutely Essential Guide to Erotic Breast Massage

Michelle Tallia

Copyright (C) 2014

The Absolutely Essential Guide to
Erotic Breast Massage

The specialized breast massage discussed in this book can give a woman more pleasure than she can imagine. If her lover is unavailable to pleasure her this way, women can easily give themselves Extreme Pleasure Breast Massage, and the great news is it's something women can do to themselves for the rest of their lives.

There are a great many positions a woman's body can be in to receive this specialized and very sexually arousing breast massage. For this example though, let's have her sitting up and at least topless. Do note however that as she gets more and more aroused, she'd probably prefer to be naked so one or both of you can access her pubic area with fingers or toys while she's getting Extreme Pleasure Breast Massage.

For this position the massager sits behind her and up against her back. If it's okay with who is getting the massage, I suggest the massager be naked as many women will lose control at some point when getting Extreme Pleasure Breast Massage and be anxiously reaching behind their lower backs to play with the massager's privates. If a woman has never experienced this type of erotic massage before, she in particular may react with callous abandon.

Before placing yourselves in any of the massage positions, you'll need to have readily available a good supply of quality lotion, massage oil and/or hair conditioner. If using lotion, try to use some brand of non-desensitizing lotion. (Most lotions put desensitizers in them to dull the pain of dry skin and other irritations. These desensitizers can at least partially desensitize breasts thus cutting down on the breast's capacity to provide pleasure. Baby lotions at dollar stores sometimes are good ones to try but lotions tend to vary by brand. Another possibility to try is a thicker hair conditioner.) Cold lotion, massage oil or hair conditioner on breasts can provide an unwelcome jolt so if warming is necessary, warm the lotion/oil up ahead of time. You can also rub blobs of it in your hands to warm it up. Always have an ample amount of this massage oil or lotion nearby as well as well as small towels to wipe the oil/lotion off of your hands and her breasts after the massage is over.

Put a sizeable glob of massage oil/lotion on each of your hands, rubbing it all over your hands to spread it out, as well as warm it if it's not yet warm. Then put your well lubricated hands on her breasts, but not yet on her nipples and areolas! That is because those provide the most pleasure and thus the best is saved for last!

It is so important that the massager make sure to keep his/her massaging hands very well lubricated. When the oil or lotion is breaking down, the massager will feel stickiness developing. The rule of thumb is that you can't lubricate your hands and her breasts too much! Do note, it can cause irritation to the skin if it's not lubricated enough.

Also the massager needs to make sure his/her nails and skin of their hands are smooth. Trim and file your fingernails and that kind of thing, to as short and smooth as possible. Otherwise she (the person receiving the massage) might feel them as they rub against her sensitive skin. She can even get hurt by them because as she is in the thongs of ecstasy, she might not realize that they are hurting her, so make sure to watch out for her and take care of this situation.

Typically the massage will provide three levels of pleasure.

(a) Massaging the fleshy part of her breast (but not massaging her areolas and nipples) should give her pronounced and very welcome pleasure; (of course the faster her breasts are massaged, the more pleasure she'll get.)
(b) Including her areolas in the massaging will increase her pleasure a lot.
(c) But massaging her nipples and areolas at the same time will really get her going.

The following (and not in order of importance) are suggestions to optimize the breast massage.

* Start from the bottom of her breasts (where the breasts meet her torso) and work your way slowly higher up to just below her

areolas. You can move your hands at varying speeds but typically the faster you massage the more pleasure she'll get.

* Simultaneously circle her boobs with each hand. Start out by using limited pressure on the breasts while utilizing only one finger, then gradually work your way up to utilizing all your fingers. Go clockwise then, counterclockwise (or vice-versa.) Remember, leave her nipples and areolas alone as much as possible until she's practically (or literally) begging for you to massage them. Sure you will "bump" into them from time to time as you massage around them. Those bumps will give her a delicious taste of what's to come.

* At its base, wrap each hand around a single breast then run your well lubricated hands around and along that breast in a steady spiraling motion up the breasts in the direction of her nipples, until you reach the edge of her areolas. Of course you can go in the opposite direction also (starting from just below her areolas and working your way down to where her boobs meets her torso.)

* Place one hand on the base of one breast; the back of the hand should be facing her head. Put your other hand on the base of her other breast, the back of it should be facing her legs. Slide your well lubricated hands from left to right and then vice-versa, across and along both breasts.

* At its base, take each breast in a well lubricated hand and with increasing speed pull up from the base of her breast to the nipple until your fingers reach the edge of the areolas (or if you're already playing with her areolas and/or nipples, go all the way to her nipples.) Then do the opposite and slide your hands back down from the top of her breasts to the breast's base (where you started from.) Repeat this procedure many, many times.

* Tease her by sliding only your well lubricated fingertips over her breasts, wiggling your fingers.

* Instead of the above, perhaps for a minute or more, you'd like to start the festivities by teasing her breasts by only briefly touching them here and there using only the tips of your fingers.

* Concentrate your efforts on only one well lubricated breast; wrap both hands around it, kneading it, pulling it and twisting it.

As previously discussed, it's strongly suggested that you take your time before playing with her areolas and then nipples. This is because she will still get a good deal of pleasure from having the 'areola and nipple-less' massage. I for one require that she even beg you to play with her nipples--because as we know this is where the breasts offer the most pleasure. I would suggest waiting until she is already well stimulated. You may stroke her anticipation by whispering in her ear that you're about to play with her nipples, then suddenly do it. She may scream with delight as an orgasm overcomes her.

Playing with her nipples is typically the high point of her massage. She'll likely be getting the most pleasure now. (Again, the faster your well-lubricated fingers move around her nipples, the more pleasure she's likely to get.)

Okay massagers you now have a choice, you can immediately start massaging her nipples fast and hard, driving her crazy, or start massaging them slowly, then progressively massaging them faster and faster until she screams in ecstasy. If you're going to massage them fast immediately, as is the first option, many women will start their orgasm then (if they haven't already.)

Don't forget you can have her use a vibrator on herself as you massage her and thus it's suggested you keep a vibrator within arm's reach. Believe me she'll find it if it's there.

As noted previously, because so often the woman you're massaging will get so aroused from all this that with both hands she'll instinctively reach around her lower back to play with the massager's pubic area. She then will not have a free hand to use the vibrator on herself. Of course both your hands are busy giving her Extreme Pleasure Breast Massage. A way to counter this is to secure a vibrator with white medical tape (the type used to hold gauge and cotton to cuts etc.) over her most sexually sensitive pubic area. (Perhaps it would be helpful if she keeps her panties on for extra support.) If you do this, more women will orgasm while you are giving her this massage.

Remember guys her nipples can get tender after orgasm and need to be left alone for a bit of time. Also don't over massage her nipples and areolas or they can get raw.

As is obvious, ladies, you can give yourself Extreme Pleasure Breast Massage in the privacy of your bedroom.

After the massage, ladies your breasts tend to become firmer for a while and often they'll feel quite good for hours.

The following is another way of giving this massage, (told from the perspective of the kinky dominant massager.) Warning it is kinky!

We will go to the bed (if we're not already there.) I will set the bed up so I am sitting with my back against the headboard of the bed and you are laying in front of me face-down on cushions with your head positioned so you can easily suck on my penis and play with my scrotum using your tied-together hands.

Also I'll put a roughly 3' x 3' sheet of plastic under your upper body to keep the massage lotion or oil from going on the bed covers. (More on this massage very soon!)

Perhaps I will also tie your bound hands to the headboard. If I do that though I will make sure there is enough slack in the rope for your hands to still move freely around my penis and scrotum while you suck. If your hands are tied to the headboard, I will be sitting on the rope as my butt will be in-between your bound hands and the headboard which your hands are tied to.

Your breasts will now be positioned, thanks to these cushions, literally just above the ground. As you suck on my penis, I will generously lubricate (and keep lubricated,) your breasts with some brand of preferably non-desensitizing lotion, massage oil or conditiner. I will warm the lotion/oil up ahead of time or rub it in my hands to warm it up, if warming is necessary. I will then massage your breasts. (Many lotions put desensitizers in them to dull the pain of dry skin. These can at least partially desensitize breasts thus cutting down on the breast's capacity to provide pleasure.) I will continue for a long time to massage your lubricated breasts as you suck on my penis. (Remember to always keep the massager's hands well lubricated!)

Using a yardstick type implement, I can reach across your back and spank you as you suck on my penis. Obviously one should make sure the woman can handle being spanked while sucking. Most can depending on the intensity of the spanking and how hard she's already orgasming.

The End

This book is sold and/or distributed with the understanding that the publisher and author is not engaged in rendering legal or other professional services. **This book and its subject matter are for entertainment purposes only.** In this publication there may be inadvertent inaccuracies including technical inaccuracies, typographical inaccuracies and other possible inaccuracies. **The writer and publisher of this publication expressly disclaim all liability for the use or interpretation by anybody of information contained in this publication.** The author, publisher and distributors of this publication hereby disclaim any and all liability for any loss or damage caused by errors or omissions resulted from negligence, accident, or any other causes. If legal advice or other expert assistance is required, the services of a competent professional person in a consultation capacity should be sought. Products, services and websites' content vary with time. Please verify any published information.

Book #3 - Special Things To Do During 3 Hours of Sex; A Step-by-step Guide

Copyright (C) 2014

Please note that the following sexual experience has kinky overtones to it. If you find any of that disconcerting, please use alternative aspects of this sex scene. This is written from a male dominant perspective.

Special Things To Do During 3 Hours of Sex: A Step-by-step Guide

Just a quick bit of information about my lovemaking style, I am a sexually dominant, heterosexual male. I need my lady love to be able to orgasm-on-demand, or agree to be trained for it. Typically she's trained to have extremely long orgasms versus several comparatively shorter ones. This is part of where my sexual dominance comes in. My lover will need to start her orgasm quickly, and continue it for as long as I am sexually stimulating her by using my hands or other parts of my body. Fortunately the human female body is built to have long, frequent and powerful orgasms, though so comparatively few women get to enjoy their incredible built-in capacity for pleasure. The truth is that orgasm-on-demand is a remarkably easy thing for women to do once properly trained.

Most men concentrate on a woman's body to stimulate her sexually, (which in and of itself is not a bad idea) but in so many cases that's not enough. I have found that most men do not adequately sexually stimulate their women's minds.

There is a natural tendency by women to be the more submissive sex during sexual activity, and that would certainly be required for the 3 hour playtime we're discussing. (Please note that if this tendency toward submissive behavior is not true in your case then this type of orgasm on demand training likely won't work too well with you.)

In her now sexually aroused state, it's normal for her subconscious mind to be more susceptible to suggestions regarding sex. People like me take it a step further and require her to do more than that during her sexual submission, specifically she will be required to orgasm long and hard, no ifs, ands or butts. Thus it is no longer her decision on how hard and long to orgasm but her lover's and I for one will require her to orgasm relentlessly.

Another way to look at it is that after being trained for orgasm on demand, the woman no longer is the one making the decision as to when she is going to have her orgasms and/or how intense the orgasm will be. She has yielded that responsibility to her lover and her mind fully accepts his/her authority in the matter.

Let's remember, a woman's subconscious mind doesn't usually care who tells it to begin orgasming, it can be her own mind giving the order or it can be her lover's. As a woman you just have to be in the right frame of mind to let it happen.

For 3 hours of sex it is very helpful if the man lasts a long time and/or is capable of getting hard frequently and with minimal downtime.

I last an extremely long time, usually for at least the whole 3 hours. I also have a thick penis which of course is a help.

Incidentally if someone is looking for an easy to find penis desensitizer cream, over the counter hemorrhoid cream under the tip of the penis can work well. I would urge the man to test it out on himself before being with a woman as if too much is used he might not even feel the stimulation enough to get hard! The man needs to know just what the right amount to use is and chances are it's a small amount.

I wanted to note that the dominant sexual position discussed in this book works best when the woman is no more than somewhat overweight.

Here are specifics of what we'd do in our 3 (or more) hour playtime.

1. When you enter my (our) place, you will take off your shoes and go kneel on the thick padding next to my bed (or other agreed upon spot like a chair or couch). Unless told otherwise, your eyes will be looking at where my midsection would be when I sit down in front of you. You will wait for me there (unless of course I'm already there.)

2. I will come over and sit in front of you (assuming I'm not already there.) I may or may not have clothes on. You'll then put your hands on my upper legs, massaging my legs with anticipation. Keep your hands high up on my legs, massaging my legs but you may not touch my penis until allowed to.

3. I will kiss you, touch you, play with you, talk to you and undress you as you kneel in front of me. At some point I may tell you to stand up and take the rest of your clothes off.

4. You will partially or fully undress me when I tell you to. When you pull my pants and underwear down, you know what will pop out!

5. I will then let you suck on my penis. You will first likely have to beg for it though. Also, remember to always play with my testicles while you suck…always!

Rule: Never let any of my penis' ooze go to waste. You know good it tastes! Beg me to let you check for ooze often! Keep sucking my ooze down until I tell you to stop.

6. Soon I will reach down and play with your exposed, vulnerable breasts as you suck on my penis.

7. At some point I may tell you to stop sucking my penis. If so I will then tie your hands securely together.

8. I may tell you to suck on my penis again or we will go straight to the following:

I will sit further back on the bed (or couch/chair) and you will lay stomach down across my lap. I will give you a nice sensual spanking, playing with your body as I do.

I will then tell you to get up and we will go to the bed (if we're not already there.) I will set the bed up so I am sitting with my back against the headboard of the bed and you are laying in front of me face-down on cushions with your head positioned so you can easily suck on my penis and play with my scrotum using your tied-together hands. If I do that though I will make sure there is enough slack in the rope for your hands to still move freely around my penis and scrotum while you suck. If your hands are tied to the middle of the headboard in this manner, I will be sitting on the rope as my butt will be in-between your bound hands and the headboard that your hands are tied to.

9. I'll also put a roughly 4' x 3' (though it can be larger) sheet of strong plastic under your upper body to keep the massage lotion or oil from going on the bed covers. (More on this massage very soon!)

Your breasts will now be positioned, thanks to cushions, so the bottom tips (which will likely be the nipples) of the breasts are just above the bed. As you are lying down and sucking on my penis, I will **generously** lubricate (and keep lubricated,) your breasts with some brand of preferably non-desensitizing lotion or massage oil. The longer the lotion can stay viscous, the better. If warming is necessary (which it most likely will be,) I will warm the lotion/oil up ahead of time or rub it in my hands to warm it up. I will then massage your breasts as you suck on my penis and play with my testicles.

I will continue for a long time to massage your lubricated breasts as you suck on my penis. (This is known as "Extreme Pleasure Breast Massage".) **Remember massagers, <u>always</u> keep you're your hands well lubricated!**

Massager and massagee will quickly notice that the nipples respond with the most pleasure from this type of massage. The massager will find that massaging his lady's breast's large fleshy area first for a while will be quite pleasurable to his slave but it is still not near as pleasurable as briskly massaging her nipples with a circular twisting motion that lets the fingers slide firmly over the nipple, not actually twisting it.

I will first make my lady beg to have her nipples massaged using this Extreme Pleasure Breast Massage technique. My lady has no more than 30 seconds to start her orgasm when I first start giving her Extreme Pleasure Breast Massage. Once I start massaging her nipples, she will have to orgasm a lot harder or risk being punished.

Using a yardstick type implement, I can also reach across your back and spank your bottom as you suck. Obviously one should make sure the woman can handle being spanked while sucking. Most can depending on the intensity of the spanking and how hard she's already orgasming.

Optional: After doing this massage for some time, you may wish for the lovely lady to be turned over on her back, her hands still tied to the bed. The man can then eat her. The lady should plan on providing her man with a lot of pussy juice. Should she not provide you with enough pussy juice, feel free to turn her over so her bottom is facing up, and give her a good spanking. Then try eating her again. (Before playing it is important that the lady keep her pussy clean and fresh.) After you've had your fill of her pussy juice, both of you can go back to the original position mentioned in this section or move on to #10.

10. At some point, I may also tie each foot to its corresponding corner of the bed. Instead I may tie your feet securely together and then tie them to the middle of the bed frame at the foot of the bed. Don't worry guys, the placement of a woman's vagina on her body while she's laying on her stomach is such that you still most likely will have easy access even with her legs closed. (However this could be a problem depending on how overweight she and/or he is.)

11. At some point I will order you to stop sucking by saying "head up". I may then get up and give you another spanking as you lay tied down, just for good measure. If you've been a good girl and are getting a lot of pleasure from all this, and if you beg for it, I will put a special vibrator (or two) inside and/or on you and set it up so it stays in place. (Tight underwear and white first aid fabric tape often work best where there are pubic hairs in the area.) I will then return to my original position on the bed and you will

continue sucking me and I will also continue giving you Extreme Pleasure Breast Massage (which I promise you'll enjoy immensely!) I will continue to periodically spank you with a yardstick type implement as described earlier.

12. After a while, I will tell you to stop sucking. I'll then clean the lotion off your breasts with a small towel(s) and remove the small plastic sheet that caught lotion that came off your breasts and my hands. I'll also remove the cushions from under you that kept your breasts literally an inch above the bed. You are now comfortably laying face down on the bed but now without the cushions and plastic under you. You still however are tied down to the bed as you lie on your stomach. (You may wish to put a clean towel under her breasts if they are still a bit oily from the massage.) I will remove any vibrators on and/or in you, as well as whatever was holding them in place. You will be completely naked, tied down, vulnerable and ready to be taken.

13. I will come back in front of you and order you to suck on my penis again. After it is hard, I will dry it off (it must be completely dry for the condom to stay on) and put a condom on it. I will then lay on top of you, stomach down, and enter you with my thick penis.

14. As I take you, you will orgasm for as long as I order you to and orgasm as hard as I order you to. You are required, as part of the orgasm on demand training, to start orgasming within 5 seconds of me entering you. Believe me, it is much easier than it may sound. You will need to ask for permission to start orgasming though! As long as you start asking for permission within 5 seconds of me entering you, you are doing fine. Of course you will need permission to stop your orgasm also! There is the possibility that at some point I will order you to stop your orgasm during our lengthy playtime (or obviously you may have to do that due to unexpected events like the kids coming home early.) If you can however, you are welcome to keep orgasming, even though direct sexual stimulation has temporarily stopped. Once direct sexual stimulation of your breasts and your vagina restarts, you'll of course have to re-start your orgasm once again (assuming it had

stopped,) and within 5 seconds as always. (Many of the ladies I have trained will continue orgasming for minutes after physical sexual stimulation has stopped.)

15. As I take you, you will orgasm for as long as I order you to and orgasm as hard as I order you to. Believe me young lady, I require long, hard orgasms from you.

16. As you know I am taking you while both of us are on our stomachs. My stomach of course is on your back. This is far and away the main position I will take you in for the entire time I take you. I may also take you doggie style depending on how overweight she is. There will however not be an emphasis on multiple sex positions during our playtime.

RULE: while I'm playing with you, if you are lying on your stomach and if I ever say "elbows" you are to raise your chest enough so that the tips of your lovely breasts are just above the bed, thus making it easier for me to play with your breasts by sliding one or more of my hands under your chest as I am taking you.

(I think you'll find that my stomach on your back position to be a very good one. Depending on how heavy and/or tall the guy is, you won't have any trouble breathing as my weight is well distributed over your bone-protected pelvis. You won't have to deal with my breathing on your face or you being pounded against the headboard like in the missionary position. Also I can hold you tightly as I take you and easily talk to you as my mouth can be right by your ear.

17. At some point I will slide one or both of my arms under your underarm(s) and put my hands on or around your hands. I can now securely hold you down with my hands. You can now reach my hands (as they are on your wrist, forearms or hands) and kiss them should that be our desire.

18. Sometimes while I am taking you like this, I will spank you. This is accomplished best by me holding myself up with one

hand/arm while I am in you and then spanking you with a paddle or the like with the other hand.

19. Often I will hold you down while I take you. I will order you to struggle FROM THE WAIST UP to get free as I am holding you down and taking you at the same time. We will do this one or more times during our long playtime.

20. Sometimes I will take you faster than other times. You will get even more pleasure from this as most any woman would.

21. Sometimes I will thrust into you as deep and hard as I can. You will get even more pleasure from this as most any woman would.

22. This is an excellent sex position for a lady to be taken anally. Perhaps she should have her anus lubed in the beginning when she is originally laid in place incase her man decides to take her anally.

RULE: Remember, the man must always wear a condom when taking her anally and he **can not** re-enter her vagina unless his pubic area has been thoroughly cleaned. A bladder infection is just one of the problems she can have if one doesn't abide by this essential safety tip.

Remember, if something is hurting young lady, you need to tell your man immediately so he can stop.

Well so there are the sexy details of how to play for 3 (or more) hours! Have fun!

The End

This book is sold and/or distributed with the understanding that the publisher and author is not engaged in rendering legal or other professional services. **This book and its subject matter are for entertainment purposes only.** In this publication there may be inadvertent inaccuracies including technical inaccuracies, typographical inaccuracies and other possible inaccuracies. **The writer and publisher of this publication expressly disclaim all liability for the use or interpretation by anybody of information contained in this publication.** The author, publisher and distributors of this publication hereby disclaim any and all liability for any loss or damage caused by errors or omissions resulted from negligence, accident, or any other causes. If legal advice or other expert assistance is required, the services of a competent professional person in a consultation capacity should be sought. Products, services and websites' content vary with time. Please verify any published information.

This book may make note of or be linked to other websites which are not maintained by any party or parties involved with this book and/or its website (should it have one.) The writer and publisher of this book expressly disclaim all liability for the use or interpretation by others of information contained in this or hyperlinked Web sites listed in and associated with this book.

Anal stimulation runs the particular risk of spread of disease and all anal activity/penetration requires a high degree of sanitation, before, during and afterward.

Book #4 – The PS-Spot Orgasm: Don't Wait Any Longer For This Kind of Pleasure

Michelle Tallia

Copyright (C) 2014.

ps-spot.com

It took three tries but it finally happened, my first PS-Spot orgasm, and I want a lot more.

— Jennifer Wilkie, Coopertown, TN

-

When my boyfriend told me about the PS-spot orgasm I didn't believe it but after some research I agreed to give it a try. I hasn't changed my life but it is nice.

— Emma Freedman, Glenwood, AR

-

It finally got me to enjoy anal sex. I'm grateful for that.

— Sara Jones, Davenport, WA

-

My husband's magic fingers have given me a lot of PS-spot orgasms.

Gina K., Galveston, Texas

-

"My husband found my PS-spot and I orgasmed so hard I passed out."

— Molly Sanders, Winston-Salem, NC

Many women know what Perineal Massage is. Women often do this (or have it done to them) to lessen the physical trauma of pushing their babies out of their vagina. Perineal massage involves massaging the perineum (the area located between the anus and the vagina.) This practice is most often done during the final weeks of pregnancy. It protects against tears to the perineal during childbirth.

This book however is about a different perineal activity.

Learning how to stimulate the female Perineal Sponge (or *PS-Spot* as it's often called) could provide an amazing treat for everybody involved. The PS-Spot can extend an orgasm, make orgasms happen quicker, make them more intense and even create an orgasm on its own.

The PS-Spot is an often overlooked part of the female sexual anatomy and definitely worth investigating. If you're a man, knowing how to stimulate it (or even knowing of its existence) can really impress a woman. If you're a woman, as you have one, congratulations! Now let's put it to work.

Connected to the amazing clitoris is a network of nerves and blood vessels that branch into various clitoral structures. These include the spongy erectile bodies: *the clitoral bulbs, the urethral sponge and the perineal sponge.* The woman's spongy erectile bodies aid intercourse by absorbing her blood like a sponge which increases their size thus pushing on the vagina walls making her vagina a tighter fit for the penis. (If one or more of a woman's spongy erectile bodies aren't working properly, it may be noticeable in intercourse as her vagina might not be as tight of a fit as expected. (This however is not thought to be a wide-spread problem.)

The Perineal Sponge (PS-Spot) is found in the lower genital area of women. Via nerves it's connected to the clitoris. It lies a little beneath the perineum (the area between the vaginal opening and the anus.)

At its top the shaft of the clitoral system divides into two 'legs' that curve downward and look somewhat like a wishbone. These are called "crura", the Latin word for legs. You cannot see or feel these 'legs' but the perineal sponge is connected to the clitoral system largely via these. The *Urethral Sponge* and the *Perineal Sponge's* connection to the nerve endings of the clitoral system via the crura helps it provide sexual pleasure. (The urethral sponge is discussed more in depth further on.)

Both males and females have a *Perineal*. In males, it's located where the penis starts (*which is located above the scrotum and called the bulb of the penis*) and the anus. In females, it's found between the vagina and anus, about 1.25 centimeters from the anus if you start your measurement from the vagina.

As both sexes become sexually aroused, our bodies create substances that cause blood to rush to the genitals, where the blood expands specialized erectile tissue called "bulbs". Men have a single bulb (the bulb of the penis) and women have two bulbs beneath the inner lips of her vagina. If unaroused, normally you can't see or feel the bulbs, but as you're aroused they expand and the genitals are suddenly puffed out, creating the female clitoral erection and of course the male erection.

The perineal sponge is internal and positioned an even distance between the vagina and anus. It's just beneath the perineum. As already noted the perineal sponge consists of female erectile tissue. When a woman is sexually stimulated, it fills with blood and becomes enlarged just as a man's penis and a woman's clitoris does during arousal. As it becomes swollen with blood, it compressing the outer third of the vagina creating a tighter fit and thus additional stimulation for the penis. (The *Urethral Sponge* does the same thing but at a different location of the vagina.)

As a general rule, if a woman knows how to find her G-spot, locating the PS-spot could be easier as the PS-spot is on the opposite side her vagina, roughly across from her G-spot.

The PS-Spot can also be stimulated through the anal canal. If you're a fan of anal sex then it's suggested you make a particular effort to stimulate PS-Spot during anal sex. Some or more women who orgasm during anal sex may be doing so largely from having their perineal sponge stimulated. These orgasms may be accompanied with ejaculation and may feel similar to orgasms from G-spot stimulation.

A description of the PS-spot comes from sexuality educator Ashley Manta. "If you take your tongue and feel the skin on the roof of your mouth, right behind your {front} teeth, that's what the {stimulated} perineal sponge feels like. It's a little firm, with ridges."

One way to look at it is that women have the G-spot on the roof of the vaginal canal and the PS-spot on the floor of the vaginal canal with the nerves of the clitoris running along side of each.

Note that the PS-Spot is not the same as the "P-Spot" as the P-spot is short for "Prostate Spot" and thus obviously associated only with men, (where the PS-Spot is associated only with women.)

It has been reported that some Tantric sex followers refer to the PS-Spot as the "Cali spot".

How to Stimulate the Perineal Sponge and have a PS-Spot Orgasm

The PS-spot is innately erogenous tissue with a large number of nerve endings. It can be stimulated by either separately stimulating the vagina or separately stimulating the rectum (anus), or by stimulating both at the same time.

A number of methods can be incorporated to achieve (or at least attempt to achieve) your PS-spot orgasm. You can use fingers, a variety of toys, particularly curved end toys, curved end vibrating toys, a penis, or a combination. The PS-spot may also be sensitive to massage/pressure when applied directly to the outer perineum (the area between the vagina and anus.)

Most often however the woman has to first be sexually excited to get the desired impact from PS-spot stimulation. First get aroused then start the PS-spot stimulation.

PS-spot stimulation can be accomplished by masturbation or by a lover.

▶ There is an online videoclip explaining how to find the PS-Spot at www.orgasmarts.com/ps-spot (Orgasm Arts). Please note, it shows naked female genitalia, so only look at it in private. The writer and publisher of this book are not associated with this graphic but very informative videoclip.

Often it's best to simultaneously stimulate the PS-spot from both top and bottom by using well manicured, very clean fingers and/or toys in both her anus and vagina at the same time.

For simplicity, let's start with accessing the PS-spot by only using one of those entrances at a time.

1) Often, *well manicured, very clean* fingers, or very clean curved-tip toys, are best for attaining sexual pleasure from the perineal sponge, (her PS-spot). This is compared to intercourse, though many women get PS-spot orgasms from intercourse.

2) Many of the same suggestions for stimulating the G-spot holds true for stimulating the PS-spot, except the PS-Spot likely is not as

far into the vagina. To find the PS-Spot using this method, since it's located across the G-spot in the vagina, (though not as far in,) just reverse the location of the pressure/vibrating force.

As the PS-Spot is located across from the G-Spot (which is located 2-3 inches in from the front of the vagina on it's roof,) an option for finding it can be to insert a curved G-spot vibrator or other toy into the vagina as you normally would to stimulate or find your G-spot, but instead make sure to turn it upside down. First though let's first have a quickie lesson on the G-spot.

To look for the G-spot, insert one or two fingers in the vagina with your palm facing her vagina. Gently bend your fingers towards you so that they stroke the front wall (thus the upper wall if she's laying on her back) of her vagina. You may feel a raised spot or series of ridges, or you may feel nothing in particular. The woman may find this extremely pleasurable, or have an urge to urinate, or both. Stroking this area with varying degrees of pressure will most likely tell the woman if she's got a G-spot or not.

To find the PS-Spot using this method, since it's located across the G-spot in the vagina, just reverse the location of the pressure/vibrating force.

The G-Spot, or Grafenberg Spot is named after its discoverer, a German gynaecologist called Ernst Grafenberg. It's defined as a bean-shaped area of the vagina that when stimulated, can lead to strong sexual arousal, powerful orgasms and female ejaculation. It's sometimes referred to as the *Goddess Spot*. 1940s research into the female orgasm led to the discovery that the female's urethral tube, which lies on top of the vagina, is surrounded by erectile tissue similar to that found in the male penis. When the female becomes sexually aroused, this tissue swells. In the G-spot zone this expansion results in a small protrusion through the vaginal wall that protrudes into the vaginal canal. It's this raised patch that is, according to Grafenberg, "a primary erotic zone, perhaps more important than the clitoris." {That is something he has been proven to be wrong about.} He explains that its significance was lost when the 'missionary position' became a dominant feature of human sexual behavior as there are other sexual positions that are far more efficient at stimulating this erogenous zone (the G-spot.)

The term "G-spot" was not used by Grafenberg himself, he called it "an erotic zone", which actually is a better description of it. Unfortunately, the modern use of "G-spot" as a popular term has led to some misunderstandings. Some women mistakenly believe that there is a 'magic sexual pleasure button' that can be activated at any time to get great pleasure. The truth is that the G-spot is a sexually sensitive patch in the vaginal wall that protrudes slightly only when the glands surrounding the urethral tube have become swollen. In other words the woman needs to be significantly sexually stimulated first to get it to do that.

For a while the establishment denied the existence of such a thing. Sexual politics had reared its ugly head. (Remember this was in the 1940s and 50s. Women back then still weren't expected to get great pleasure from sex and many questioned whether a vaginal orgasm was even possible. They tended to believe a clitoral orgasm was possible though.)

There have been reports of women undergoing 'G-spot enhancement'. This involves injecting collagen into the G-spot zone to enlarge it (push it further into the vagina so it interacts with the thrusting penis more.) According to one source, "One of the latest procedures to catch on is G-spot injection. Similar substances to those injected into the lips to plump them up can now be injected into your G-spot. The idea is that this will increase its sensitivity and so give you better orgasms."

A significant number of women are getting enhanced sexual pleasure and/or orgasms by stimulating the area where the G-spot is suppose to be but there remains a major controversy as to whether the G-spot exists. The writer of this book assumes the G-spot exists but has no conclusive proof.

This is one of the suggested ways to find your *G-spot*. Make sure you're quite sexually aroused. Insert one or two pulsating fingers (a vibrating curved tip toy may work better) two inches into the vagina and starting at the top of the vagina, exert the necessary force, or vibrating force, at the 12 o-clock position. If your G-spot doesn't make its presence known, try repeating this process further in another third of an inch, then another third of an inch and then to play it safe another third of an inch and another third. If it hasn't made it's presence felt yet do the same procedure but starting from two inches in at the 12:30 position and if necessary the 1:00 position. If the G-spot remains hiding try this procedure in the 11:30 position and the 11:00 o'clock position. There of reports of women finding their G-spots in the 10:00, 10:30, 1:30 and 2:00 position. Again you want to test from two inches into the vagina (1 ½ inches to play it safe) and then further and further into your vagina. Most G-spots, if they're found, are found 2-3 inches in from the front of the vagina, but yours might be located outside those parameters. Please note that you may be one of the hundreds of millions of women that don't have a G-spot and there remains some doubt in academic circles as to whether it really even exists. Assuming it exists, it's located in the vicinity of the urethral sponge (which we'll discuss more about later) not the perineal sponge.)

In 2011, researcher Adam Ostrzenski claimed to have found the first evidence of G-spot anatomical structures by dissecting a cadaver in Poland. Between the fifth and sixth layer of the vaginal wall, there were grape-like clusters Ostrzenski believes are erectile tissue that would function as a G-spot. The research was published in The Journal of Sexual Medicine in 2012. Critics of Ostrzenski's claim note that he provided no evidence that his sample consists of nerve endings, that the structures play a role in arousal, or that they would be in one specific area. Ostrzenski said that part of the reason he did not detail a precise type of tissue and how it works is because the Polish regulations that govern dissection of fresh cadavers prevented him from taking samples for histological testing. He said that he is not suggesting that the G-spot he reported to have found will be in the same place, or have the same effect, for every woman.*

*(Healy, Melissa (April 25, 2012). "Doctor says he's found the actual G spot".) (Taken from http://en.wikipedia.org/wiki/G-spot).

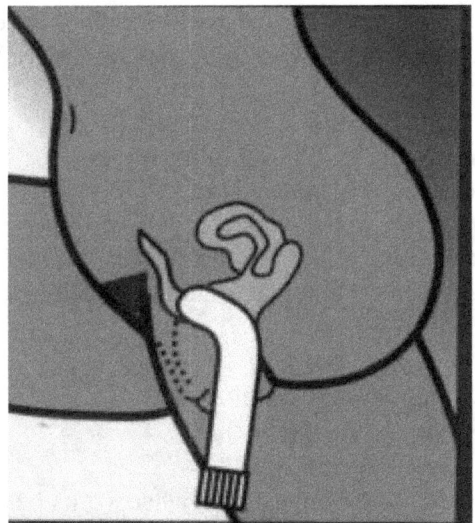

Positioning of the G-spot Vibrator

Locating and/or stimulating your PS-Spot via the vagina

If a woman is lying on her back, the *back (posterior)* wall of the vagina is the part of her vagina that is closest to the bed, and the *lower* part of her vagina is the part of her vagina that's closest to the vagina's entrance.

As the PS-spot is erectile tissue, typically the woman needs to be turned on for it to be most significantly activated (filled with blood and thus 'erect'.) By activated I mean getting firmer to the touch. This can be accomplished in the usual manner, through breast stimulation, clitoral stimulation or even kissing depending on how quickly and easily she gets sexually stimulated. In other words in many cases it doesn't work as well to start playing with her PS-Spot if she isn't already turned on.

When only using the vagina, (versus using both the vagina and anus) the PS-spot can be accessed via the *lower back* wall of the vagina. It's between ½ to 1½ inches into the vagina. Your *well manicured, very clean* finger or toy enters the vagina and <u>pushes down</u>. Start by pushing down only a half inch in, then a little further in until she feels the stimulation. (Typically it's not more than 1½ inches into the vagina.) You flick/move your finger in a manner that gives her the most pleasure. If you're using a toy perhaps sliding it back and forth a bit will do the trick, particularly if it's a vibrating toy.

2) If a woman wants to try to stimulate her perineal sponge during intercourse, either with a penis or dildo, she should position herself in a manner that directs the phallic implement of choice toward the back (thus bottom if she's laying on her back) wall of the vagina. Three recommended sexual positions are:

- The missionary position
- The woman-on-top position
- Seated and facing each other.

You want to do the opposite of what works best for targeting the G-spot. For instance doggy style is a good G-spot sex position but not as good for the PS-spot.

Locating and/or stimulating your PS-Spot via the anus

The rectum lies against the sacrum (lower backbone) in a gentle curve down to the anal opening which as you know is penetrated during anal sex. The front (anterior) wall of the rectum and rear wall of the vagina, and the thin layer of tissue between them, are together called the *rectovaginal septum* (or wall).

Anally the perineal sponge can be accessed via the front wall of the rectum. (If a woman is lying on her back, the *front wall* of the rectum is that which is closest to her vagina.)

Use a *well manicured, very clean finger* (perhaps a thumb so you can enter her vagina with the index finger at the same time but remember to keep anything that has touched her anus, away from her vagina.)

▶ There is an online videoclip explaining how to find the PS-Spot at www.orgasmarts.com/ps-spot (Orgasm Arts). Please note, it shows naked female genitalia, so only look at it in private. The writer and publisher of this book are not associated with this graphic but very informative videoclip.

As the man's prostate is stimulated from being taken anally (as that's his *P-spot*), conversely a woman's PS-spot can be stimulated from being taken anally.

The reason the G-spot feels good when touched is because it stimulates the clitoris from the clitoris' underside. The clitoris isn't just what you see on the outside. It actually goes a couple inches inside of you.

The PS-spot is located closer to the rectum than the G-spot, though further from the clitoris. Remember though that the PS-spot is connected to the powerful clitoral system thanks to its physical connection to the clitoral system via the clitoris' "crura" (leg-like nerve growth.)

1) When testing to see if a woman has a PS-Spot, it's likely first best to explore for, and/or stimulate the potential PS-spot with a thinner sex toy or normal size finger. Length should be a problem as it's located ½ to 1½ inches in. A wider sex toy, or a penis, should the receiver not be used to it, can cause physical anxiety and/or trauma that takes away from the PS-spot sexual enhancement experience.

2) Generally speaking, fingers or curved-tip toys are best for applying pressure on the perineal sponge, whether insertion is occurring via the vagina or via the anus. In many cases though, simple insertion by a penis into the anus can have more success stimulating the PS-spot than simple insertion by a penis into the vagina. Chances are good that if a woman orgasms from anal sex alone, at least part of that is from PS-spot stimulation.

As previously noted the PS-Spot is located between the rectum and vagina so when insertion of a toy or phallus is occurring in the anus, the emphasis needs to be on the part the rectum closest to the vagina.

3) While taking a woman doggie style or the like, push the penis or dildo toward the front (bottom) of her body (meaning her stomach, pubic hair, face etc.).

Locating and/or stimulating your PS-Spot by utilizing the anus and vagina at the same time.

This is the preferred way to search for and activate her PS-Spot. Remember anything that touches the anus can not touch the vagina.

1) The woman should be sexually excited so the erectile tissue including the perineal sponge has filled or is filling with blood. This makes the PS-spot easier to find and more sensitive.
2) Use plenty of lubricant.
3) Use a *well manicured, very clean finger to* enter her vagina and another finger/thumb to enter her anus at the same time.
4) Massage, rub and/or vibrate the PS-Spot simultaneously from both the top and bottom holes. The PS-Spot is located only ½ to 1½ inches in.
5) Just because she didn't orgasm from it this time or not get a great deal of pleasure doesn't mean she won't when you do it again in the future.

If having intercourse, one of the parties can stimulate the unoccupied hole.

The Perineal Sponge may respond to pressure from outside of the perineal body

The perineal sponge may respond to pressure from outside the body too, though this could depend on how much fat and muscle is in between it and your skin. Try a vibrator that you would normally use on your clitoris and press and move it against the skin which is located equally between the vagina and anus. Chances are good pushing up will help. With experimentation you can determine the best way to stimulate the PS-Spot this way, or if your PS-Spot can even can be stimulated that way.

Stimulating the Urethral Sponge

The perineal sponge is not the same as the urethral sponge. Like the perineal sponge the urethral sponge is a spongy cushion of erectile tissue found in the lower genital area of women. It is however located across the vagina from the perineal sponge. It sits against both the pubic bone and vaginal wall, and surrounds the urethra. Its job however is much the same, with sexual stimulation, engorge itself with blood and make a tighter more pleasurable fit for the penis. It however is closer to the clitoris.

The G-spot is located in the urethral sponge and one theory is that as the urethral sponge engorges itself with blood from sexual excitement (as does the perineal sponge), thus getting larger, it pushes down on the G-spot area thus activating the G-spots clitoral nerve connection, giving it's host sexual pleasure.

The Urethral Sponge provides women with the "U-spot". The U-spot can be located in different parts of the Urethral Sponge; its size can vary from woman to woman. (Unfortunately many women don't have a pleasurable U-spot to start out with.) The U-spot isn't the same as the G-spot.

The urethral sponge encompasses sensitive nerve endings connected to the clitoris. It can be stimulated through the front wall of the vagina. Some women experience intense pleasure from stimulation of the urethral sponge (U-spot) while others find the sensation irritating. The urethral sponge surrounds clitoral nerves, and since the two are so closely interconnected, stimulation of the clitoris may stimulate the nerve endings of the urethral sponge and vice versa. Some women get U-spot pleasure from the rear-entry position of sexual intercourse (whether she's laying on her stomach or on her hands and knees) as the penis is often angled slightly downward and can stimulate the front wall of the vagina, and in turn the urethral sponge.

If you have a pleasurable U-spot you want to get to know it better as there is documented evidence of women also getting earth-shattering orgasms from it as women have with the PS-spot.

Conclusion

Women, enhance your sexual pleasure with a part of your body you already have and likely are not even using!

Is the PS-Spot also one of your hotspot spots? I certainly hope so and for many people it is. (Incidentally if the G-spot isn't a hotspot for you, don't assume the PS-Spot won't be also, as actually often it is.) Unfortunately there's no guarantee that optimal utilization of any sexual part of your body it will make you scream like a ban chi. The important thing is that you explored an erroneous zone in your body (and there are others) to make sure you could be all you can be.

► There is an online videoclip explaining how to find the PS-Spot at www.orgasmarts.com/ps-spot (Orgasm Arts). Please note, it shows naked female genitalia, so only look at it in private. The writer and publisher of this book are not associated with this graphic but very informative videoclip.

Guys, an easy, cheap way to delay ejaculation for those special occasions is - anti-hemorrhoidal and anesthetic ointments. I know a man who used NUPERCAINAL for that purpose. It's an over-the-counter medicine and readily available at many drug stores. I suggest however that you only put a little on, particularly on the underside of the tip of the penis. It will be absorbed by the skin after a while. *Guys you'll have to test it yourself to see what the best amount for your use is because if you put too much on you might not feel her stroking you in an attempt to make you hard.* Please note this disclaimer. I do not know if there are any side effects to it's use and though I know of nobody having a problem with it, it's possible. Contact a physician before using it or doing something like it. Sorry but I don't want to risk getting in deep do-do with the American Medical Association or any other official organization.

The End

Absolutely Essential Tips for Buying & Selling On eBay

Important Tips for Buying on eBay

1) Last Minute Bidding Frenzies - Perhaps you've noticed that often there's a bidding frenzy in the last one minute of bidding. New bidders may suddenly start bidding in the hope that the previous bidders will not be watching or can't increase their bid in time. Often however it's because of *Sniping*.

Sniping websites automatically bid on your behalf, often in the last 10ish seconds. Simply sign up, enter an eBay item number and the maximum price you're willing to pay. Hidbid.com and goofbid.com offer sniping services that place bids for you.

Typically you'll need to give sniping sites your eBay password for them to work (ugh!!) Obviously that is a serious security concern.

There's little protection from eBay if things go wrong when sniping, since you willingly gave your password to a third party. If you do sign up for such a service, never use the same password for eBay as you use for other accounts like banks accounts or email addresses.

2) Second-chance Auction Scams, Beware of Them - Unscrupulous people sometimes watch bidders in high-dollar auctions and try to take unsuspecting buyer's money after an auction ends.

The scheme, known as a *Second-chance Auction Scam*, is just one of many types of Internet auction frauds reported to the *Internet Crime Complaint Center, or IC3*.

Second-chance scammers wait until auctions end and then offer bidders that lost, a phony second chance to purchase the item -- usually through a wire transfer service. This happens more often than people realize, beware!

3) Misspelling Search Tool - Typojoe.com, goofbid.com, bargainchecker.com, fatfingers.co.uk and baycrazy.com - There are many items listed on eBay every day that have misspelled words in the title. It's unfortunate for the seller but chances are good those listings will not come up well in eBay's search engine (because misspelling causes keyword problems) and thus not bring the seller top dollar. Their loss can be your gain!

4) Bidding Tip - Often sellers start auctions at .99 cents, (or at least under a dollar) hoping a bidding war will erupt. Many items go unspotted, staying at this super-low price (99 cents). *LastminuteAuction.com* hunts for eBay auctions due to finish within an hour but where the price still is very low.

With these items in particular, double-check delivery charges, as some sellers hope to recoup costs by charging a little extra (though eBay's now set maximum delivery charges for many categories).

5) Don't Forget About Facbook - Facbook Marketplace is a force to be reckoned with. Also sellers often are open to haggling. Just log on to your account at Facbook and search for "Marketplace". It's also worth checking to see if there's any local Facbook selling groups in your area.

6) Nigerian Type Scam for Paying. These unscrupulous people want to pay with a money order that they claim to already have handy. Often it's for more than the purchase amount. He writes to ask if the seller would be "honest enough" (or something of that nature) to send him the extra cash along with the item. (However he might just try to only buy the item with it and not ask for extra cash.) Unfortunately the money order can look okay but is counterfeit. They particularly like the *Buy It Now* feature.

7) Set Long-term Alerts For Rare Items - If you want something very specific or hard to find, set a 'favorite search' and eBay will email each time a seller lists your desired item.

Simply type a product in eBay's search bar, such as "silver dollar", and click 'save search'. Be as specific as possible for the most accurate results. When (and if) someone lists one, you're alerted with an email.

8) Don't Assume eBay's the Cheapest Place To Get Your Item -
Many people assume that if it's on eBay, it's automatically the
least expensive place to get it, but that often isn't the case. Perhaps
you'd also like to use *shopbots* (shopping robots) that check
numerous Internet retailers to find the best price. Type into a
search engine "shopping comparison sites".

The same rule applies when buying used merchandise. Check used
marketplaces on Amazon.com and Play.com - you may even get it
for free on Freecycle or Freegle.

9) Check the eBay Going Rate For an Item - There's a quick way
to check an eBay product's average price. Enter the item into the
search box and click "completed listings". What will come up is a
list of prices that similar auctions have already settled on. After
that, sort it by "Price: lowest first". If the price is red, it means no
one bought it. Green means it sold. Figure out the average price.

*10) eBay has banned the selling of intangible items, and that
includes curses!* - Among the items that were prohibited as of
August 30, 2012, are "advice; spells; curses; hexing; conjuring;
magic; prayers; blessing services; magic potions; healing sessions;
work from home businesses and information; wholesale lists, and
drop shop lists."

11) Haggling on eBay Can Pay Off - There's nothing wrong with
asking for a discount, even if the listing doesn't have the "make
offer" indication. Haggling works best on *Buy It Now* listings, or
auctions with a high start price and no bids. Also you'll likely do
better if you haggle as the auction is coming closer to closing as
the seller could start feeling more desperate.

To contact the seller, click on the seller's nickname then "ask
seller a question". If you're polite, you'll likely get further. Blunt
requests such as "dude, how about $15?" likely won't work out as
well. Remember the seller is likely going to lose money doing this
so no point in being annoying.

Once you've arranged a deal, try to keep the transaction within eBay. Ask the seller to add (or change) a Buy It Now price. That way you don't lose the usual eBay buyer protection privileges.

12) Other Things to Do To Exploit Sellers' Screw-ups - Some sellers make basic mistakes, leavings goods going for bargain money.

As well as spelling boo-boos, another error is to leave out key details such as shoe size, dress brand, saying a console's an a Wii when the photo shows a Xbox. At this point, many buyers give it up as "too much hassle".

So contact the seller to fill in gaps, but don't ask the question via the item's listing page, (because that way, when the seller replies, eBay lets them add their reply to the main listing, so it's no longer your secret.)

Instead, ask the question via the seller's profile (make it clear which item you're talking about). They might not bother with the extra hassle of adding it to the listing, so you'll be the only one in the know.

Also the seller might not realize how pricy an item he/she actually has.

13) Tool to Track Down Crazy End Times - Listings that finish at anti-social times often get fewer bids, thus sell for less. To locate auctions that finish when fewer people are around to bid on them, use BayCrazy's *Crazy End Time* search. (A lot more on the best times to end your auction in the next section of the book "*Selling on eBay*".)

Check out their auto-bidding tools if you don't want to spend all that time in front of the computer bidding at odd times. Other BayCrazy.com tools include "unwanted gift" and "ending now" searches.   www.baycrazy.com/search.php?page=nightowl (Baycrazy offers other eBay related opportunities also.)

14) Search Descriptions as Well as Titles - eBay automatically searches seller's titles for results that include your specified keywords. If you're not getting the results you want, try also searching the item's *description* too. (To do this go to Advanced Search.)

For example, imagine you were searching for a REI Jacket. Unfortunately the seller may be selling one but only put "Ski Jacket" in the title however he mentioned "REI" in the description. Include description in your search and then it should then come up.

15) Search Using eBay Boolean Logic - If a seller could describe an item different ways, you can make eBay search for several different ways of describing it at once. Just place "((" at the beginning and enter different phrases individually enclosed by quotation marks, then followed by commas.

So for example, type... (("fishing tackle", "hook", "reel" ...and it will simultaneously bring up listings that contain the words "fishing tackle", "hook" and/or "reel".

16) Add A Few Extra Cents to Your Bid - When bidding, you enter a "maximum bid", and eBay makes automatic bids on your behalf up to your maximum bid.

Don't enter a round number. For example, if a coat is currently selling for $20, and the most you are willing to pay for it is $25, enter a maximum bid of $25.24. If someone tries to outbid you by entering the round number of $25, they will receive an outbid notice. eBay will go your bid, even though it's just 24 cents more.

17) Be Somewhat Skeptical of Feedback - eBay sellers have a feedback rating that acts as a useful guide to previous seller's opinion's of them. As a guideline, look for a seller with more than 98% positive feedback and a high feedback score of at least 30. Also ensure you read their feedback from their *selling*, not just their *buying*. (To see their feedback, click on their username).

18) Seller with Zero Feedback Could be Cause For Concern - Think twice before purchasing expensive items from a seller with zero feedback.

Remember feedback's useful but not infallible. One thing to watch for is traders selling a number of cheap things for $1ish each to build their feedback, and suddenly listing items costing hundreds each.

19) Check to Make Sure You're Bidding on the Actual Item - Sometimes you assume you're bidding for an item on eBay (or any auction site,) when all that's actually being sold is a link to another site selling it. People are not suppose to be able to sell these on eBay but they can fall through the cracks.

Always read the whole description in detail before bidding. Often the catch is hidden in the text at the end – an attempt to protect the seller from any recourse.

20) Scam - Beware of it - It's a red flag if a seller writes "Before bidding, contact me" then asks for a money transfer. Thieves who hijack actual eBay accounts might use this tactic.

21) Scam - Beware of it - Always be worried if you're asked to pay by an instant money transfer service such as Western Union or MoneyGram. Instant money transfer payments cannot be traced and are highly popular with thieves.

22) Sneakily Find Underpriced Buy It Nows - Feel free to hunt for Buy It Now bargains also. Perhaps the seller under-values their item making their price a good deal.

These steals are snapped up quickly. Go to "Advanced Search", select a category you're interested in, filter it to show *Buy It Now* items and sort the results.

23) Always Complain within 45 Days - Under eBay's buyer protection program, 45 days is the most number of days you have to open a case if you're unhappy with your purchase. (There are

some exceptions such as tickets for events that are months away.)
Read more on eBay's protection policy.
http://pages.ebay.com/help/policies/buyer-
protection.html#conditions1

Under eBay's own Buyer Protection rules, buyers are eligible for a refund if the item's "not as described", meaning it didn't match the seller's description. http://pages.ebay.com/coverage/index.html

24) Pay by PayPal - Avoid sending checks and never use money orders. It's much harder for scammers to disappear with your cash when you use eBay's online payment system, PayPal.

Paying this way costs the same as paying by check, but means you're covered by eBay's Buyer Protection program. If an item is faulty, counterfeit or non-existent, you are far more likely to get a refund.

25) Outbid? Don't Give Up On It Yet - Missed out on a desired item by pennies? Don't give up hope. As every seller knows, sales sometimes don't materialize when buyers change their minds or can't come up with the dough. Because of that feel free to send a friendly message such as: "Hi, I've been looking for this poster for years and just saw your finished auction. Please let me know if the sale doesn't come through."

They may send a *Second-chance Offer*, which are sent out by sellers to unsuccessful bidders if the winner fails to pay up. Ask them to relist at an agreed *Buy It Now* price.

26) Know Your Consumer Rights - When buying from a person who makes or sells goods for resale on eBay you often have the same rights as when buying in person from a shop that does the same. This means your goods must be of satisfactory quality and as described.

With private sellers it's buyer beware. Buyers' only rights under law are that the product is fairly described and the owner has the right to sell it.

Under eBay's own Buyer Protection rules, buyers are eligible for a refund if the item is "not as described", meaning it doesn't match the seller's description.

27) Beware of All The Fakes - While eBay has a 'flag and remove' policy to help identify fakes, still plenty fall through the cracks.

If you're buying big-name brands, do your research first. Carefully check sellers' feedback and post on the forum's eBay board to get others' opinions. Be especially wary of overseas sellers or branded items that seem especially cheap.

The more *unprofessional* the photos, likely the better. Thieves often take professional photos from the brands' sites. Legitimate sellers typically take photos of items at home that might not come out as well.

28) Think Twice Before You Give A Seller Negative Feedback - Of course, negative feedback is often justified but have a heart, don't leave negative or even *neutral* feedback without first trying to work the issue out with the seller. Most sellers are good folks who will try to help particularly, as it can mean a lot to their business to stay in your good graces.

Remember eBay users can view the feedback you've left for others, and if you leave a significant amount of negative feedback, they may well decide you're too high of a risk to sell to.

29) Add An Item You're Interested in to eBay's "Watch List" - Want to keep track of an item without bidding on it? eBay lets you add items to a "Watch List", so you can relax knowing you'll get an email reminder within 36 hours of the auction ending. To watch an item, just click the *"add to watch list"* link in the upper part of the item's eBay webpage.

30) Don't Do Private Purchasing - Sellers may suggest you do a deal outside eBay for a cheaper price. If you do you'll likely have less protection if things go bad. You won't be able to leave negative feedback and you won't be protected by eBay's Buyer Protection Plan.

31) Think Safety When Picking Up An Item In Person - The usual precautions apply. If you get to their door and the seller's holding a butcher knife, now's the time to run.

32) Think International - There's bargains to be had on overseas eBay sites. To include foreign auctions in search results, click "worldwide" for location.

Still can't find what you want? Another option is buying directly from *international* eBay sites. The main ones are USA, Canada, Australia, Germany, France and Spain - there's a full list at the bottom of eBay's homepage. Make sure that the item reads *"Shipping to: worldwide"* before bidding as some international sellers only do business with their country's buyers.

Always factor in postage and if applicable, custom fees. Remember that return postage fees could be hefty.

Also what kind of credit card protections will there be? You're often still protected by eBay and PayPal's buyer protections (if you use PayPal), but it's worth investigating. Type in "buyer protection" in PayPal.

33) Don't Forget The Online Classified Ads - Again, let's not assume that because it's on eBay, that's where you'll get the best price for an item. Unfortunately that's often just not the case. Type "top classified ad sites" or something of that nature, into search engines. There's also *Freecycle* and *Freegle*. (Those two sites offer free stuff. freecycle.org and ilovefreegle.org.)

Remember, anyone can post on these classified ad sites. If someone asks you to pay by MoneyGram or Western Union, as always be concerned. It's a bad way to pay.

34) Check Other Auction Sites Also - There are other auction sites that can be found through search engines. If you're searching for something specific, it's also worth adding it to your search. *Auctionlotwatch*.com is a useful shopbot for online auctions. Search for an item and it trawls the big auction sites for you.

35) *Check Cashback and Voucher Websites* - Check cashback websites to see if there's money back available on your eBay purchase. Type into search engines: "cashback and voucher sites".

Cashback sites give you a cut of their proceeds by setting you up with product and/or service providers.

36) *eBay has trained teachers that could be in your area.* Also see eBay University. Check out:

http://pages.ebay.com/sellerinformation/howtosell/university.html

Important Tips for Selling on eBay

1) Join eBay Forums - Ask questions about anything, selling, buying etc. Great information is posted already and could be of use. Work together as a team. Find eBay and other auction forums by looking those up in search engines. Ebay has forums also. http://forums.ebay.com/category/Ebay-Discussion-Boards/2001

2) eBay Research Tool 1 - To help in your research about selling items, you can go Type into a search engine "best selling eBay items." EBay provides that information.

3) eBay Research Tool 2 - You can use Ebuyers (www.ebuyersedge.com) to just search eBay for items as well as set up a saved eBay search (or a number of them). You'll get alerted with an e-mail when a matching item is listed.

4) Sell Refurbished Products - Refurbished products fall somewhere in between new and used products. Refurbished products are not new, but often they aren't significantly used either. Sometimes a customer buys the product and for whatever reason, returns it for a refund. The item is then returned to the manufacturer, given an inspection, repaired as necessary and sold as refurbished.

There are various ways an item can become refurbished.

1. The packaging of an item can be damaged during shipping. In that case the item is sent back to the seller/manufacturer. Refurbished items usually come with manufacturer's warranties. Although sometimes the warranties that come with refurbished items are for a shorter period of time, the products are usually in very good condition.

2. Items that have a slight defect or flaw, like a scratch or mechanical flaw, might be returned to the manufacturer. The manufacturer repairs the items, repackages them and marks them refurbished.

3. Demonstration units are also considered refurbished, but generally that's when they're returned to the manufacturer, inspected and repackaged.

4. Brand new overstock items can also be marked refurbished.
5. Sometimes it's a situation where only the packaging of an item is opened. It's re-packaged or even just closed up and marked as refurbished.

Refurbished Products Advantages:

a. Refurbished products are significantly cheaper than new products. They also come with warranties, boxes and everything else new products come with.

b. Selling refurbished products is more profitable, even though refurbished products cost significantly less than new products. On eBay (and at other places) refurbished products can sell for the same price as new ones. (Many people buy refurbished products thinking they're buying new ones.)

c. Refurbished products are sometimes new! When you buy a lot of refurbished products they might actually be overstock items or factory overruns. In that case you would be buying new products at a fraction of the price.

Refurbished Products Disadvantages:

a. Refurbished is not new, even though refurbished products can be exactly the same as new ones, people simply prefer new items.

b. Refurbished products are sometimes the previous year's models. If you're selling electronics or computers it could bring the selling prices down.

5) Finding Products To Sell - Unfortunately finding products to sell can be the toughest part of starting your eBay business. Many people end up opting against starting an eBay business because they can't find a good supplier.

a) YELLOWPAGES.COM - www.yellowpages.com. Try this first. Yellowpages.com can find specialized suppliers in your area. Type in "wholesale" into the search box and you will be given a bunch of subdirectories to further explore. Make sure the search is based on a location near you. Next type "wholesale directory" or "wholesale directories" into search engines.

When searching also try inputting keywords such as overstock, salvage, surplus, liquidation, auction, refurbished, refurb, supplier, closeout, wholesale, etc.

b) BUY FROM AN ACTUAL EBAY SELLER. Buy multiple items and get a discount. That discount could be your margin of profit.

c) BUY WHOLESALE LOTS FROM EBAY AND RESALE THEM - Go to eBay and search for "wholesale lot". If you buy a big lot, you could find you profit best by individually selling the items in the big lot.

d) PERHAPS SELL DIGITAL COUPONS. You should be able to get them for free. As of this writing, people are posting that coupons sell well on eBay. If you're selling coupons, you need to mention that your auction is for the time you spend finding, assembling (sorting) and sending the coupons to the buyer rather than selling the coupons themselves. It's illegal to sell coupons and that's why auctions say the payment is for the time to gather and sort them. Still it can take time to find good coupons and first folks need to know where to look.

e) BUY FROM LIQUIDATION COMPANIES - A liquidator is someone that buys overruns from big retailers (Sears, K-mart, Wal-Mart etc.) at a fraction of the wholesale price. Sometimes big stores can't sell everything they have. The stuff they couldn't sell needs to be gotten rid of as soon as possible to make room for new products. This is where liquidation companies come in. They buy the overruns products, often at a fraction of the wholesale price. When a liquidation company buys a couple of truckloads full of overruns, the next thing it must do is sell these overruns ASAP to make room for more overruns. Since the liquidator must get rid of the products as soon as possible, the products are sold at cheap prices and often in bulk. Perhaps there are liquidator stores in your town what would make you a deal and you wouldn't necessarily have to buy in bulk.

f) BOOK SALES - With books, you can sell a digital product that can simply be emailed to your customer. No packing and shipping involved! Selling books on eBay is easy. In fact there are systems you can implement to essentially automate the entire process. You could do a *Buy It Now* auction, or just start the bidding at a reasonable price. When the auction ends and the buyer pays you, all you need to do is email the book to them. Again, that's the great thing about downloadable information products: no packaging or shipping is necessary. Perhaps you'd like to offer an entire collection of books to sell on eBay. You'll need books that you own or have given you resale rights.

g) You can sell peoples' houses, cars, boats, or even jewelry collections. Just look in the for sale listings of your local newspaper and look at all of the great stuff for sale that would sell on eBay. Call up the owners of the items advertised in the newspaper and offer to sell the stuff for them. Looking for stuff in newspapers is great because the people that are using a newspaper to sell something probably know little about eBay and are desperate to get rid of the stuff they're advertising. These people are also the ones that are willing to lower the price and haggle, and that is great because the lower the price they are willing to let the item go for, the more profit you can make by selling their stuff.

h) RUNNING ADS TO FIND MERCHANDISE - You can run ads in print media and/or post what you're looking for in Internet forums with something like "I will buy your stuff". As previously noted, if you are going to use this method you will need to pick a used product that keeps its value well. If you're going to use this method you should buy things like jewelry and watches, antiques and other things that appreciate with age.

A previous seller's success story was selling old collectable Apple computers. This is a type of item that some people have laying around in the basement or attic, and will likely never use again. They're more than happy to unload it and get a little money for it at the same time. But on eBay it was a whole new ballgame. There are thousands of people who collect old collectable computers.

6) Sell To Resellers - Anyone looking to buy products and resell them to make a profit is a very good customer that will come back and buy from you again and again. Plenty of people buy stuff on eBay then resell it on eBay! There are also those who buy products on eBay to resell them on their other ecommerce websites or actual stores they may own. A lot of PowerSellers (special higher volume eBay sellers with a closer relationship to eBay) started by buying stuff off of eBay and simply putting it back up for auction.

7) Order Samples If Possible - This is a particularly good tip if you don't have a chance to inspect and see the products you are ordering in person. Many people starting out on eBay make the mistake of placing a big order before actually seeing what they're ordering. By ordering samples you'll be able to test not only the quality of the products you're ordering but the service, communication and legitimacy of the company you're ordering from. If you're thinking of selling designer clothing on eBay, be extra careful when ordering your supplies from the Internet. There is a lot of fake (counterfeit) clothing being sold on the Internet. Remember the pictures on the supplier's website may look real, but that doesn't mean they will be sending you what's in the picture.

If you find a great deal but the "supplier" won't allow any sample orders and wants you to pay through an untraceable method, be wary.

8) Second-chance Offers - If the buyer of your item falls through, you can send the other bidders a *Second-chance Offer* to see if they're still interested in buying it.

9) The Listing's Title - The title of your listing should be clear, relevant to what you are selling and attention grabbing. Always include the correct spelling of the item in the title. Don't try to make the title "cool" by deliberately misspelling words, unless perhaps if the slang name for it is popular. If you misspell the title, your listing won't show up in search results because presumably most people aren't searching for the slang name (or misspelled version) of the product.

The title has to be short (eBay rules), so make sure you include the name of the item and abbreviated descriptions, and try not to waste any space on words that are not needed. *By the same token, always use the entire allotted space to write your title. In general, the longer the title, the better, as long as all your keywords are relevant.*

10) Keywords & Relevancy - Make sure the brand name of what you're selling is in the title! If you're selling a Champion Portable Generator, your listing title should include the make and model number, in this case "New Champion 42431 Portable Generator, 1500 Watt". Your listing title should be a short, abbreviated description of the item you are selling.

The name of the product in the title has to do with the search results (keywords). If people want to buy your portable generator they may search "portable generator, generator, Champion, Champion portable generator," etc. You want to make your listing show up in as many search results as possible.

In review, a wild but catchy title will definitely grab the attention of most people who see it, but won't come up in many people's search results, unless also in the title listing is the name of the product that people would type in when looking for it. (Even that's not guaranteed to work.)

11) If a potential customer wants other people's opinions on a product you sell, you might want to send them to the Amazon.com's webpage for the site as Amazon posts feedback from buyers of that same product. Make sure that Amazon is not selling it for less than you are or that idea could backfire!

12) Mention Flaws: If there is a flaw in the item you are selling, make sure you mention it (though try to call it something else like "scratch" or "mark" if that's what it is.) If your product has a flaw and you don't mention it in your listing, you could get negative feedback and a request for a refund from the person who buys the "flawed" item.

If possible, make the flaw sound positive. You could say "this product has a small dent that has no effects on its operation, but because of this you save big bucks!"

Mentioning a flaw also can make you look like an honest person. You can even have the flaw mentioned in your bullet points - Small scratch on the top (saves you money!!)

13) Host Your Own Pictures - You can host your own pictures on another website or your eBay Store and thus show many, many more photos free of charge.

14) Payment Options: - You should offer the customer several different choices of payment. Most of your customers will pay you through PayPal, (PayPal is owned by eBay,) so make sure you get a PayPal account (www.PayPal.com). Of course, not everyone who buys items on eBay prefers PayPal, some may prefer Western union's Bidpay or another payment system. Another one you should sign up for is StormPay as it can be used by people in some countries where PayPal is not used or as popular. For your free StormPay account go to: stormpay.com.

Wire Transfers - Unscrupulous overseas buyers prefer these as they're not as traceable. It's preferable not to take them.

15) Offering SquareTrade Warranties - If applicable to what you're selling, another good way to build trust is to sign up for SquareTrade warranties at www.squaretrade.com. www.squaretrade.com/seller-faq

16) About Me Page - The About Me page is often overlooked by many eBay sellers (and buyers.) While having the free About Me page likely will not dramatically increase your sales, it can help if you have good things to say about yourself and a nice picture. Note, many sellers only include links to their listings and maybe not enough information about themselves in the About Me page.

17) People Bidding with 0 Feedback ratings - Having a good to great feedback rating is so important as you know. Many sellers refuse letting members with 0 feedback bid on their auctions. Getting a negative feedback from somebody that unpredictable is simply a risk we don't want to take. In many cases, we simply don't trust them.

18) Best Time To End Your Auction - The best time for an auction to close (end) is in the evenings and on weekends as that's when most people are on the Internet for that type of activity! You want to make sure that when your auction is closing (ending), everyone that's interested in it is available to bid on it. The mornings are the times that the eBay website gets the least visitors (as people are more often sleeping or working.)

If you live in the Eastern Time Zone, list your auction between 9pm-11pm, Central Time Zone list between 8-10pm, Mountain Time Zone between 7-9pm, and for the Pacific Time Zone list between 6-8pm. This will give you the biggest exposure at the end of your auction. The debate is out as to what day your auction should end on. Some sellers report that Tuesday, Wednesday and Thursday are best. Other sellers report that Saturday and Sunday are best.

There are a few exceptions though. For example, some business products sell best during weekdays and during work hours. Obviously this is because people are usually ordering those types of products at work, for work. Studies have shown that a listing that ends at peak hours can attract up to 25% more bids than one that ends in non-peak hours. Listing your auctions at optimal times is one of the easiest ways to attract more bids.

To end the auction in the evenings, you'll need to put the item for sale in the evening (*or use listing software [see next page] to do it for you*) as eBay considers each day to have a length of 24 hours.

Note, it's eBay's practice that when someone's auction is ending, that listing shows up higher on keyword search results (which is a good thing!)

19) Terms of Service Webpage (Yours) - That's something even a lot of experienced sellers don't seem to include, though it likely won't be necessary if all the information is already in your FAQ webpage. For instance, what's the return policy? What are the shipping options, and what will they cost? What are the accepted methods of payment? How soon is payment to be sent? What is the warranty?

20) Listing Software (For Your Items) - Listing software organizes your eBay listings making the listing part of your business simpler and more efficient. There are many different kinds of listing software. You can do an Internet search for them.

Turbo Lister is free software from eBay. Turbo Lister allows you to upload thousands of listings at a time. It saves listings, schedules your listings and uploads them to eBay automatically. Using it you can edit multiple listings at the same time, preview what your listings will look like before uploading them and more. More eBay software is offered at:
http://pages.ebay.com/help/sell/advanced_selling_tools.html

21) Drop Shipping What You Sell - With drop shipping all you have to do is list items up for auction and when they sell, you contact your supplier, who ships the products from their factory, straight to your customers. In theory drop shipping is a good way to go, but it could offer problems. What happens when you sell items and your supplier sends them to the wrong addresses? What happens when you sell items and your supplier is out of stock? In those cases your reputation suffers. If you are going to use drop shipping; make sure there is good communication between you and your supplier (drop shipper.) Also make sure you have some products in stock in case the supplier runs out by the time your auctions have closed.

22) eBay Stores - eBay stores can be great if you have a number of items to sell. First you'll need to reach the minimum number of feedbacks required (10) to open one. Most PowerSellers have eBay stores. Store sellers can see an increase in profit of up to 25% in the first three months of opening the store (according to eBay). Having your own eBay store can save you a substantial amount of money in listing fees and let you sell items in a fixed price format as well as selling via auctions. Also you can list items for a much longer time and store them in your inventory list for 30, 60, 90, 120 days and even "Good till Cancelled". You can feature links to other auctions in all your listings by utilizing a cross promotion tool. There are also bonuses like your own search engine and monthly reports from eBay featuring statistics and dada about your sales in the past month.

An eBay store also gives you a location. It gives you a base of operation, a place where people can easily find you, and a place where repeat customers can come back to. Your customers will be able to bookmark and return to your store, and it may also be indexed in the major search engines. So if you're selling silver dollars, and someone does a BING search for silver dollars, your eBay store may appear in the results along with the usual online retail websites! Obviously this can increase your traffic greatly, and likewise boost your sales.

23) Your eBay Store Identity - Ideally your eBay store should look different from your competition. You can use the design templates eBay offer you, but perhaps it's best to use original graphics. Fortunately eBay Stores are customizable. Ideally, to establish your name, your eBay store should appear like your listings as much as possible. Same colors, design and look.

24) Get a Domain Name - You need to get a simple and memorable domain name. A domain name makes it simple for people to find you. The standard web address eBay will give to your store will look like this: *stores.ebay.com/yourname*, this is not a very memorable web address and it's too long to be easy to type into a web browser. It would be best if you had a web address like *mystore.com*.

The End

www.ingramcontent.com/pod-product-compliance
Lightning Source LLC
Chambersburg PA
CBHW070813290526
45795CB00002B/712